GW00707895

INDISPENSABLE QI GONG
For People On The Go!

INDISPENSABLE QI GONG
For People On The Go!

by Joan Foo Mahony

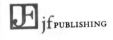
jf PUBLISHING

First published in Malaysia in 2002

© 2002 by Rhino Press and Joan Foo Mahony

The moral rights of the author have been asserted

Published by Rhino Press Sdn Bhd (Co. Reg. No 426848-A)
3rd floor, 23 Jalan 3/76D, Desa Pandan, KL 55100, Malaysia

Printed by Yang Printing Services (Co. Reg. No. 058442-V), Malaysia
Design and Layout by Noemy Zainal

A publication by Rhino Press
A catalogue record for this book is available from the National Library of Malaysia

ISBN 983-9476-12-2

CONTENTS

Chapter Seven
QI GONG FOR HEALTH AND WELL BEING

Appendix

For Terry, my 'indispensable' husband

ACKNOWLEDGEMENTS

This book is dedicated to my qi gong master and teacher, Master Mak Chung Man, a man of extraordinary talents whose compassion and commitment to this ancient art has helped me regain my health and strength. Master Mak's willingness to share his knowledge and impart some of his wisdom to me through the years has made this book possible.

This book would not have been possible without the help of so many wonderful people, and although I cannot name everyone my thanks go out to all the kind people who helped make this book a reality.

I need and wish to thank Fay Khoo of Rhino Press, who is also a good friend, for a superb job in editing and for proof reading my many drafts with great skill, patience and good humour.

I am also greatly indebted to Dr. Amir Farid Datuk Isahak MBBS (Aust), MMED (Singapore), MRCOG (UK), an outstanding obstetrician and gynaecologist who practises not only modern medicine but has effectively combined this with holistic healthcare. Dr. Amir, a firm believer in the self-healing powers of qi gong and the President of the Guolin Qi Gong Association, Malaysia, has taken time from his busy practice to write the foreword to this book.

The Wushu Federation of Malaysia, of which I am an honorary advisor, has helped me enormously. My grateful thanks, especially to Dato' Kee Yong Wee.

Last but not least are the various members of my very patient family and friends including my husband Terry, my sister Dr. Janet Foo and my nephews Nicholas and Ian Lim, and, in particular, Benjamin Foo. You were all such a great help. Among my many friends who encouraged me during the project are Olivia Wong, Judy Freshwater and Helen Tang, to name just a few. Thank you all so much.

ILLUSTRATIONS

I am also indebted to Sara Russell for the wonderful illustrations in this book. Sara was on holiday in Malaysia when I persuaded her to do the illustrations. Her approach was precisely what I wanted for the book — not stock textbook drawings but a refreshing take that is at once appealing and realistic.

Sara Russell was born in Scotland. Her foundation art course was achieved at Kingston. She attained her B.A. from Canterbury and went on to obtain her Masters degree at the Central School of Art in London. She is currently working on window displays and visual merchandising for popular sports stores in London whilst accepting private commissions. Sara also runs a children's art club from home. She lives with her husband and two daughters in London.

FOREWORD

by Dr. Amir Farid Datuk Isahak
MBBS (Aust), M MED (S'pore), MRCOG (UK)

Within the many different styles of qi gong one can achieve tranquility, health, and fitness as well as mastering the art of self-defense. In ancient times, qi gong was an esoteric art shrouded in mystery and accessible only to the most dedicated aspirants who had to become disciples to masters and monks who lived and taught in temples and monasteries.

As such, qi gong was known only to a few, and for thousands of years its practice remained exclusive. Whilst tai chi, kung fu and other Chinese healing exercises and martial arts have been widely taught to the masses and known to the west, the same is not yet true for qi gong. Many Chinese themselves still do not have any idea of their very valuable heritage.

But the situation is changing rapidly. Many qi gong masters are now teaching students who come from all over the world. In fact, many of them now teach in the west. Since most people are already aware of other Chinese arts, they should have no problem accepting and learning qi gong once it is demystified and made simple and easy to understand and practise. Everyone can get the tremendous health benefits from qi gong.

Joan Foo Mahony is a Malaysian Chinese who lived in the west for much of her life. The best modern medicine could not cure her severe osteoporosis (which resulted from unexplained hormonal aberrations), and she was forced to return to her heritage and rely on the healing power of qi gong. Needless to say, she has regained her health and leads an active and robust life whilst others her age are slowing down with menopause!

This book is a magnificent endeavour to demystify qi gong. Joan has adopted a refreshing approach by teaching the most practical qi gong exercises for people on the go with simple easy-to-follow instructions. There are no rigid rules or suffocating styles, only simple exercises anyone can do. Now you can start experiencing the benefits of qi gong without having to look for a master first. If you like the healthy changes that you will definitely get, you can of course find a good master to guide you further.

It is indeed a privilege to have known this remarkable lady, and I am sure you will find this book equally remarkable!

DR. AMIR FARID DATUK ISAHAK
President
Guolin Qi Gong Association, Malaysia

AUTHOR'S PREFACE

I first met Master Mak Chung Man under less than propitious circumstances in Hong Kong, in 1992. A jet-setting lawyer whose work took me all over the world, I was the stereotypical professional on the go, always with a few projects on the burner and living life in the fast lane. It is easy to understand, then, how devastated I was to learn (after an ice-skating accident and subsequent x-ray and bone density tests), at the 'tender' age of 43, that I had lost 40% of my bone density. I was a 'young' woman with the skeleton of an octogenarian.

Despite a battery of complicated tests in the USA, my doctors were left puzzled as to how or why my body seemed incapable of retaining calcium. I was approaching severe osteoporosis at an alarming rate when one doctor concluded that a hormonal abnormality in my glands was causing my brain to scramble messages to my blood. Therefore, no matter how much calcium I ingested and regardless how much calcium my bones contained, a message was relayed by my brain that I had "Insufficient calcium! Insufficient calcium!" This meant that my blood was constantly 'stealing' calcium from my bones which was then (because it was not needed) expelled through my urine. I remember thinking, in a moment of dark humour after one of many urine tests, that I could have built a rather formidable calcium pyramid with all the mineral I was losing.

The prognosis was not good. I was deteriorating so quickly that my skeleton would soon be unable to support the hyperactive lifestyle to which I was so accustomed. Typically, I refused to accept my fate lying down and in 1992 flew from Boston to Hong Kong, where – a firm believer in the ways of the east – I met with Master Mak. My life and my fate were effectively rewritten from that moment onwards.

Master Mak changed my life by teaching me about my body's vital life energy, called 'qi'. He also coached me in the art of healing myself through the use of qi gong exercises.

Diligent and regular practice of qi gong soon arrested the osteoporosis, whilst concurrently improving my health to the extent that I was soon able to resume my normal active lifestyle. I am now 53 years young, a whirling dervish who is constantly on the go. Although I no longer practise as a lawyer, I am actively involved in several business concerns and projects. I climb mountains, sail, snowshoe, run, play tennis, lift weights and plunge into just about any form of physical activity without a second thought. My doctors are flabbergasted at how I have managed to confound such a debilitating illness and triumph with the aid of something as simple as qi gong.

Truth be told, I do not spend hours contorting my body in impossible poses everyday. A more realistic calculation would see me allocating barely twenty minutes of my daily time to qi gong, and that's because the qi gong that Master Mak taught me is not a discipline that requires a specific time and place for it to be practised. Indeed, much of its appeal lies in the fact that it can be fitted into otherwise wasted chunks of 'dead' time, such as arduous hours spent queuing for tickets, commuting in trains, and even whilst watching television.

Partly due to my immeasurable debt of gratitude to Master Mak, and partly because qi gong works – I am living proof! - I wanted to share the benefits of qi gong with people like myself, who are harried by everyday exigencies and have no time to stop and reflect on the quality of one's life. I am by no means a qi gong master, but I have lived with qi gong as an integral part of my life for the last decade. At the very least, I know it well. With Master Mak's guidance and invaluable advice, this book has become reality, and I have him to thank for this. I hope you will find qi gong as useful and wonderful as I have.

Enjoy!

INTRODUCTION

Like many ancient eastern disciplines, qi gong has become increasingly popular in recent years and is now practised the world over, where once it was confined to the far east and a mere smattering of exponents. And while many books have been written on the subject, none provide the novice practitioner ease of reading and use in everyday situations where time is of the essence.

This handy guide has been written precisely with those two driving principles in mind. Whether at work, at play, or in moments of leisure, *Indispensable Qi Gong* aims to give readers a chance to use qi gong to optimise those little pockets of time to improve well being, both physically and mentally. A step by step guide with accompanying illustrations aim to demystify the many stances of qi gong, covering most everyday situations, so that qi gong can be done even whilst sitting in a traffic jam, for example.

Indispensable Qi Gong does not aspire to be an exhaustive tome on this wonderful discipline. It does not deal with the origins of qi gong, nor does it attempt to explain the scientific theories surrounding qi gong and how or why qi gong is a catalyst in the healing process. What it is, however, is an essential guide for novice and veteran practitioners alike. Put simply, *Indispensable Qi Gong* was designed for you and other like-minded people on the go, with busy schedules and scant time to waste. Qi gong is not complicated, because ultimately qi gong is for everyone.

Remember: you can do qi gong anywhere – in a bus, on a plane, even while playing golf. Make *Indispensable Qi Gong* your daily companion, and use its easy to understand instructions and illustrations to familiarise yourself with the stances that will eventually become second nature, to improve your life.

Remember: **you** choose which stance to practise, just as **you** also choose which stance is suited to your needs at any particular point in time. There are no hard and fast rules; practise qi gong in your own time, at your own pace and for as long or as briefly as you wish.

Also remember: you are not mastering qi gong. Far from it. However, you will become well versed with a number of qi gong stances which you will find especially beneficial for you and which you can easily do in the midst of living your busy lives. As Master Mak is fond of telling his students, "It's always better to do only one stance regularly and do it well than to attempt unsuccessfully to master eighty or more movements." Use qi gong to strengthen mind and body, to prevent and even to cure illness, and as a result, enjoy a fruitful, long and healthy life.

WHAT IS QI GONG AND
WHY IT IS GOOD FOR YOU

Although an ancient form of Chinese traditional exercise dating back to more than 3,000 years, qi gong is by no means an enigma. 'Qi' translates as the body's 'vital life energy', while 'gong' literally means 'exercise'.

Marry the words, and qi gong means the mobilisation of the internal energy in the human body. When we practise qi gong, we are effectively activating the vital life energy that is stored in our bodies to unblock and to balance stagnant qi. This in turn enables us to stay healthy. If we are sick, the practice of qi gong will assist in directing the body's qi to the affected areas and encouraging recovery.

Qi gong is about self-healing; it is something each of us can do for ourselves whenever we have a spare moment. By integrating simple qi gong stances into your everyday lives, you will notice a discernible improvement in health, strength and energy, as well as feeling more positive and calm.

If I had to summarise in one sentence why qi gong works, I would probably explain it thus: practising qi gong regularly builds on and balances the overall life energy flow in the body.

Ancient Chinese medicine holds that illness or fatigue occurs when the circulation of qi is blocked or stagnated. Hence, once we can get the qi to circulate, then the cause of illness is removed. Therein lies the fundamental philosophy of qi gong. By mobilising our inner qi and encouraging its smooth, unimpeded flow through the body, we will be able to strengthen our immune system by harnessing its own internal energy systems with efficacy.

How qi gong works is clear: qi gong reduces the body's metabolism and oxygen consumption by a third. When this happens, wasteful energy depletion is also lowered, thus effectively allowing qi or vital energy to accumulate rather than dissipate. The storage of qi or fresh energy facilitates the body's immune system, which in turn consolidates vital internal organs and helps the body to stay healthy and fight illness.

Qi gong helps us 'corral' stagnant qi into a reservoir of energy known as 'dantien' or 'field of energy'. The dantien is located about two inches below the navel. The qi "moves" first to the dantien, circulating downwards from there to the abdomen and loins. It then moves upwards through the coccyx and spine all the way to the top of the head and then down the front to the forehead. This smooth, continuous and invisible circulation of qi is the vital life energy which works to clear blockages in the body's main energy channels (also known as meridians). Meridians are invisible but because they are energy channels, one can visualise them 'flowing' throughout the body and linking one vital organ to the other. As the qi or vital energy flows through the meridians, it nourishes and strengthens all the cells that comprise each of these organs. Similarly, when one is sick, qi is channelled directly to the 'problem areas' to help the body wage war against illness. However, when one is well, smooth flowing qi prevents sickness whilst simultaneously keeping us energetic and in the pink of health.

In short, qi gong **stops** wasteful energy loss and **stores** vital energy in the body. This qi then **circulates** through the meridians or energy channels to all the vital organs. When all this is in **balance,** this promotes good health and prevents or alleviates illness. This is the essence of qi gong.

BEFORE YOU BEGIN:
A FEW HANDY POINTERS

1. Always stand solidly with both feet apart and shoulders aligned

2. Do not tense your body. Relax!

3. The mind should be tranquil

4. When you turn, the head turns with the eyes

5. Except for the stance at bedtime, do not close your eyes when practising qi gong. By keeping your eyes open, you will be – although relaxed – fully alert to your surroundings and unlikely to be unsettled by ambient noises or occurrences

6. You may not always be able to wear loose comfortable clothing since some of these exercises may literally be done on the run. However, if you are wearing a tight belt, do try to loosen it

7. The stances should all flow. Avoid abrupt jerking movements

8. There is no particular breathing method required. Breathe naturally and calmly at all times through your nostrils (not your mouth which should be closed). Some qi gong masters do instruct on the importance of a breathing technique but Master Mak believes that it is not strictly necessary. All one needs to do is to breathe naturally and slowly

9. Do not be alarmed if your fingers or palms intensify in colour and become warm when doing qi gong. This indicates that the qi is flowing

10. When qi gong is done correctly and qi is flowing well, you will feel hot and a warm tingling sensation will surge throughout your body, particularly at your fingertips. You may also experience a slight force at the fingertips and a tingling sensation always accompanies this 'force'

11. You may shake or tremble involuntarily. This is also normal when qi is flowing

12. When practicing qi gong, try not to look at red or yellow hues as these are considered fiery colours and will not relax your mind. Green is best which is why many people rise early in the morning to practise qi gong among trees and plants

THE BASIC QI GONG HEAD POSITION

Imagine that the crown of your head is held up by a string, or imagine you are carrying a pile of books on your head. Position your head accordingly, and fix your gaze straight ahead, with chin slightly lowered, back straight and with your buttocks tucked in.

ALSO REMEMBER

Your arms should always be held slightly apart from your body so that your armpits are not closed. This prevents qi being inadvertently trapped under your arms and is very important in all aspects of qi gong exercise.

AT

PLAY

a) Stand firm with your feet apart at shoulder width, arms relaxed beside your body, palms facing inwards and fingers spread

b) Swing your body and arms from the waist towards the left, keeping your right arm in front and your left behind

c) Slap your right hand on your left shoulder and the back of your left hand to your right hip

d) Your head should follow your body as it swings, remembering to fully stretch your neck by looking behind, over your left shoulder

e) Repeat this about 7 times on each side

WHAT IT DOES

Warms up your limbs for exercise. No more cramps!

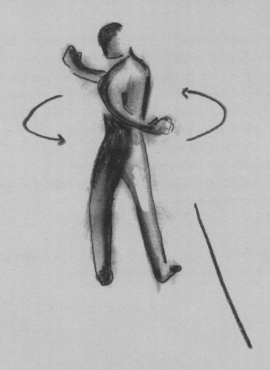

AFTER SPORT OR EXERCISE

a) Stand with your feet shoulder width apart, toes pointing forward at a slight angle. Keep your legs straight and breathe naturally

b) Making sure your arms are straight, clasp your hands in front of your tummy, palms facing downward, and your thumbs not touching

c) Keeping your hands clasped, slowly raise your straight arms – palms outwards – all the way above your head until they're fully stretched and your palms are facing the sky

d) Stretch yourself to the limit while looking straight ahead

e) Unclasp your hands and return your arms to the starting position

f) Repeat as many times as you wish!

WHAT IT DOES

Gives you a wonderful total body stretch, whilst also cooling you down and relaxing those well-worked muscles

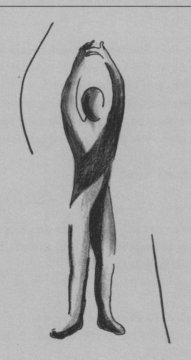

ON THE GOLF COURSE

a) With fingers spread and palms facing outwards, reach your straight arms towards the sky and, standing with your feet shoulder width apart and legs straight, bend forwards from the waist
b) Now bend your legs, placing your hands on your knees. In a continuous sweeping motion, run them up along your thighs and upper body, leaning backwards at an angle as you do so, and finishing with your arms straight and extended
c) Straighten your body and repeat

WHAT IT DOES

It's great for circulation, but also strengthens your liver and kidneys, massages your spine and supports your back muscles, thereby relieving pesky muscle pains at the waist and knees

HANDY HINT

Keen to improve your game even more? Stance vii is excellent for golfers as well, so remember to add that to your qi gong routine

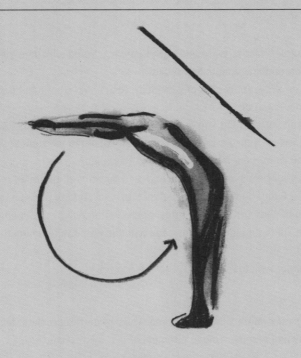

WHILST VACATIONING

a) With your left foot forward and right foot back, stand with your soles flat on the ground and weight in the centre

b) Keep your arms at the side of your body, with elbows bent and palms facing downwards

c) Now bend your left leg and transfer your weight forward, and in a flowing motion, extend your arms, palms still facing down, to the front of your body and cross your hands without touching them

d) Turning your palms upwards, still in a fluid movement, return your arms to the side of your body as you move back to your starting position (a)

e) Finish with your arms at your sides, palms facing down, and your left foot 'opened' (ie resting on its outer edge with the little toe touching the ground)

f) Now repeat with the other leg

WHAT IT DOES

Loosens your joints, opens your respiratory system, increases lung capacity **and** improves blood circulation!

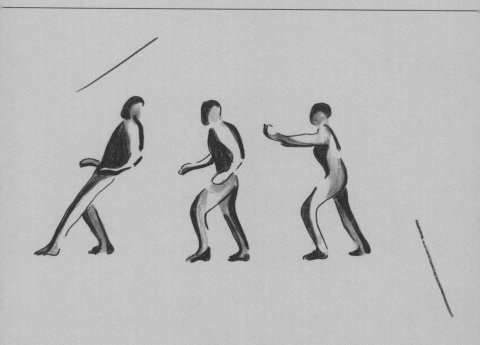

CHAPTER 4

QI GONG

WHILE

COMMUTING

IN THE PLANE

A) First Stance

a) With your head in the basic qi gong head position, sit with your spine straight and (don't cheat!) not reclining on the seat

b) Place your feet shoulder width apart and flat on the ground and rest your hands on your thighs, with palms facing upwards and fingers spread, claw-like

c) Now check that your elbows are open and your arms are not touching the sides of your body, to optimise the benefits of your qi 'workout'

WHAT IT DOES

Helps you arrive in better shape by alleviating fatigue and jet lag and promoting circulation

DID YOU KNOW..

that the open position of your elbows encourages maximum airflow because it opens the collarbone?

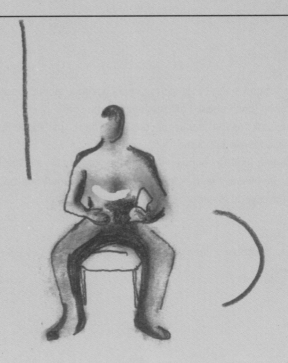

29

B) Second Stance

a) With your head in the basic qi gong head position, sit with your spine straight and (don't cheat!) not reclining on the seat
b) Rest the backs of your hands on your lower back, just above the hips, with palms facing outwards
c) Now lift your heels as high as possible, but keep your toes firmly on the ground, then lower them, repeating the lifting and lowering motions briskly for several minutes

DID YOU KNOW..

you can also prevent deep vein thrombosis when flying by doing this exercise

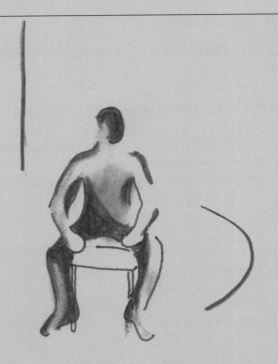

IN THE CAR

Whilst in traffic or whilst waiting

a) Raise your legs a couple of inches off the floor, keeping them straight, and flex your feet

b) Now sit upright with your head in the basic qi gong head position, and your back **not** leaning against the car seat

c) Extend your arms in front of your body, with palms facing forwards, and fingers spread, as though you're showing someone the number 'ten'

WHAT IT DOES

Relaxes your body, tones your legs, and reduces water retention. Now how about that?

DID YOU KNOW..

you can also do this exercise if you are a passenger

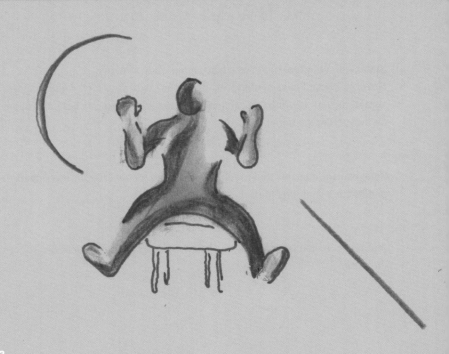

IN THE TRAIN, SUBWAY OR BUS

a) Stand with your feet apart, and your upper body straight
b) Now bend your knees slightly, resting the backs of your hands with fingers spread on your lower back, remembering to keep your arms bent and open (ie away from the body)

WHAT IT DOES

Relaxes your muscles and restores energy. It's also a great stress-buster and it tones your legs too!

DID YOU KNOW..

that this exercise is also great for golfers? Try it next time you're on the green

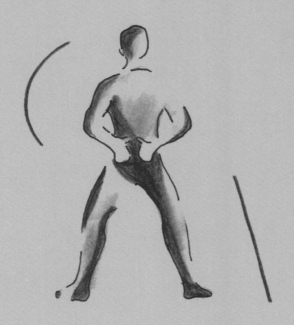

CHAPTER 5   QI GONG

AT

THE OFFICE

BEFORE WORK BEGINS

a) Stand with your feet shoulder width apart and your body relaxed
b) Extend your arms at shoulder height in front of your body, with palms facing upwards and lift your heels 1 to 2 inches off the floor
c) Now drop your heels back to the ground with a slight thud, turning your palms down towards the floor as you do so
d) Repeat this exercise 7 times only

WHAT IT DOES

Improves mental alertness and is super for jump starting the day

DID YOU KNOW..

that the thudding motion increases alertness?

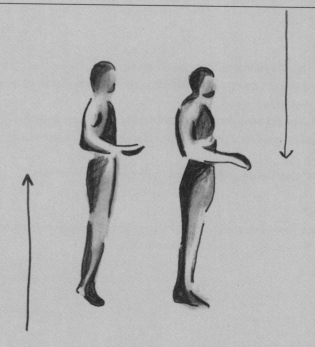

a) Stand up from your seat, and clear a space
b) Imagine you are sitting on a chair with your feet shoulder width apart and knees bent
c) Put your hands lightly on your hips, keeping your upper body straight
d) Now rotate your body from the waist clockwise in a deep circular motion
e) Repeat seven times and then again anti-clockwise seven times

WHAT IT DOES

Relaxes your neck and shoulder muscles and aids blood circulation

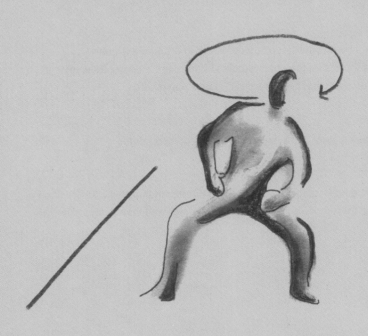

DURING MEETINGS

a) Sit upright with your feet shoulder width apart on the ground
b) Rest your arms on the chair handles (if there are any) or place your hands on the table, fingers spread, palms downwards

WHAT IT DOES

Increases mental alertness and prevents mental fatigue

DID YOU KNOW..

Chinese emperors of old used to sit in thrones in this particular position to make them more alert to their surroundings and their subjects

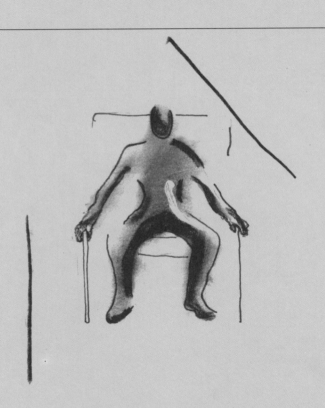

CHAPTER 6

QI GONG

AT HOME

OR DOING
CHORES

WHILST WATCHING TV

a) Don't be a couch potato! On your feet!
b) Stand with feet shoulder width apart and extend your right arm, with fingers spread and palm outwards
c) With your left arm waist high at your side, bend your left elbow at a right angle away from your body, with the palm facing down
d) Now balance on your right leg, whilst raising your left leg as high as you can, with your knee bent at a right angle away from the body, and your foot flexed
e) Try balancing for as long as you can, making sure your back is straight and you are in the basic qi gong head position, before repeating with the other leg

WHAT IT DOES

Strengthens your lower back and calf muscles

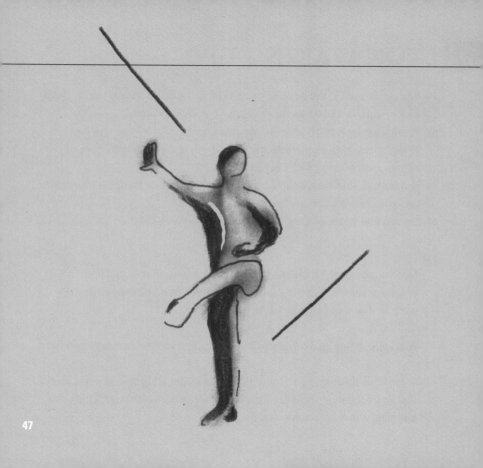

UPON WAKING UP

a) With your head in the basic qi gong head position, stand with feet shoulder width apart, relax your body and bend your knees slightly
b) Raise your arms to chest level and mimic embracing a huge oak tree. Check that your palms are facing your chest, and your fingers spread with thumbs facing up and outwards
c) Remember: your hands should **not** touch. They should be half a foot apart and your elbows must be lower than your hands
d) Do you feel warm all over? Well done, you're doing it right!

WHAT IT DOES

Rids your body of Tin Man stiffness and improves your circulation. What a great way to start your day! Practise this stance regularly and you'll find yourself a lot stronger too

HANDY HINT

This stance may also be done sitting down, but your back must be straight

DID YOU KNOW..

if you imagine that you are part of the tree under a big blue sky, you can feel yourself absorbing all the goodness of the earth. It's wonderfully life affirming and a great sensation!

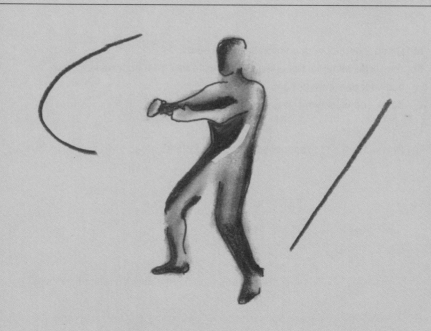

AT BEDTIME

a) Lie on your bed with your legs slightly apart
b) Your arms should be at a slight distance away from both sides of your body, elbows outward and palms down
c) Relax and close your eyes. Easy!

WHAT IT DOES

Relaxes you and prepares you for a good night's sleep

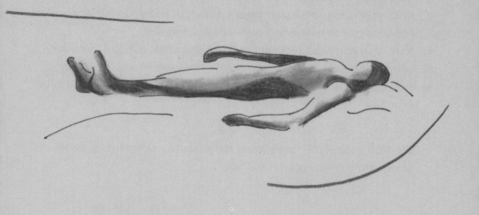

a) Lie as though in a foetal position but on your back, with your knees tucked into chest, legs at a 90 degree angle and feet flexed
b) Raise your hands above your chest – as though shielding your face – and keep your palms facing down and fingers spread
c) Now raise your head, tuck your chin into your chest and hold that stance
d) Lower and repeat the movement again a few times until you feel tired
e) Had enough? Go into stance xxiii above, and you'll be sleeping like a baby in no time

HANDY HINT

Die-hard insomniacs can try doing stance xxiii for stress before doing stance xiv to ensure greater efficacy

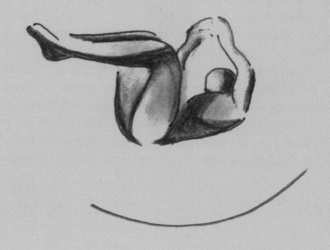

WHILST QUEUING

For Tickets, In The Supermarket, Wherever!

a) Place your feet shoulder width apart and bend forward from the waist while looking down

b) Put your hands on your knees, and – with your knees in a slight squat – mimic sitting down on a chair

c) Slide your hands up your thighs and straighten your body, then let your arms hang loosely away from your hips, as though you're a cowboy about to draw your pistols. Your palms should face inwards and your fingers should be spread, so that there is a slight force in your fingertips

d) Remember – you should be in the basic qi gong head position

e) Don't forget to relax your body, breathe naturally and not hunch your shoulders!

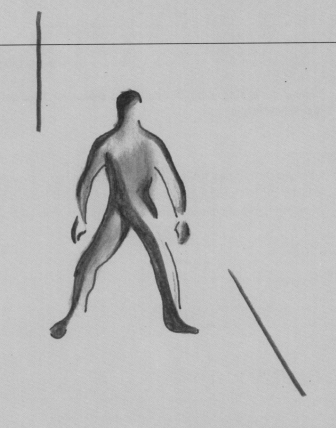

It's super for storing energy in your body and also helps you get those supermodel thighs

When your body is bent forward, your tailbone should point towards the ground so that qi can flow continuously to your belly without much conscious exertion. When done correctly, this stance will happen with very little effort at all

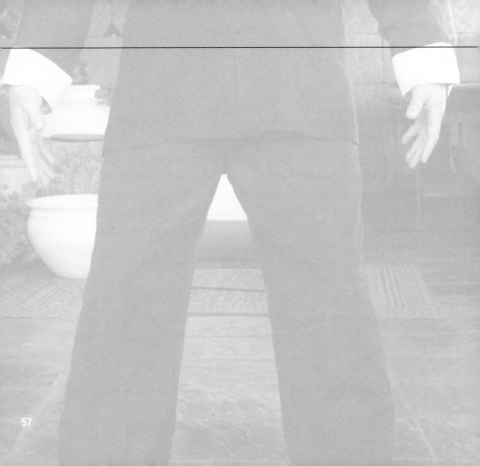

a) Stand on your left foot and place your right leg behind your body at a right angle, with your right heel off the ground
b) Your left arm should be slightly bent and next to your left hip, and your fingers should be spread with your left palm facing the ground
c) Now bend your right elbow and raise it next to your right temple, close to your ear but not touching, palm downwards and fingers spread
d) Twist your body towards the left and look all the way backwards towards your right foot for a huge stretch
e) Repeat on the other side

WHAT IT DOES

Strengthens your spine and eases tension while encouraging qi to move around your body. This stance also tones thighs, biceps and your neck

HANDY HINT

Sneak a peek at the cover photo to see how the stance is done

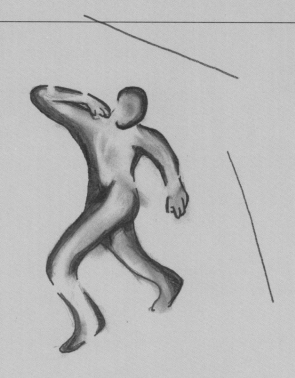

59

CHAPTER 7

QI GONG
FOR HEALTH

AND
WELL BEING

a) Stand with your knees bent and feet apart at shoulder width
b) Bend your elbows and put your hands next to your ears with fingers spread and palms facing the ground
c) Now tilt your body backwards at a 45-degree angle

WHAT IT DOES

Besides flushing out your nasty flu symptoms through sweating, it also regulates your blood circulation. Got a headache or stomachache? Say good riddance to it with this stance

HANDY HINT

Drink a glass of warm water to prevent dehydration as you will sweat profusely doing this stance, especially if done correctly

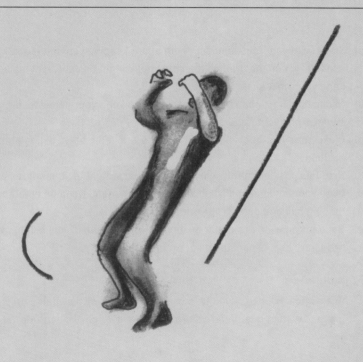

WHEN YOU'RE ILL

a) Stand with your feet shoulder width apart, keeping your left leg straight and left foot on the ground, then put your weight on your right leg and bend your right knee

b) Mimic holding a giant ball, remembering to keep your palms facing inwards and your fingers spread

c) Make sure your back is straight and you are in the basic qi gong head position

d) Hold this position for a while then shift your weight to your left leg and bend your left knee whilst straightening your right. Keep on embracing that big ball and don't drop your arms!

e) Repeat from side to side for as long as you can, whilst still holding your imaginary ball. Expect to sweat profusely

DID YOU KNOW...

this stance will cause you to 'sweat out' your flu so it's vital to drink a glass of warm water before starting to prevent dehydration

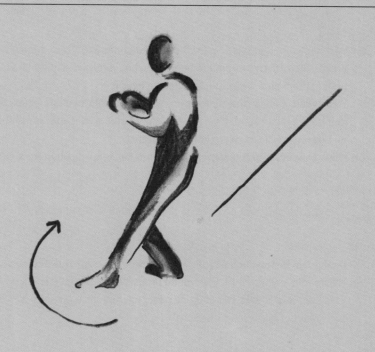

a) With feet shoulder width apart, bend your knees slightly and raise your arms – elbows away from the body – to shoulder level as though you're resting them on a high wall and looking over it

b) Your hands should resemble claws, with fingers spread and palms cupped and facing the ground. It's important to remember that your arms should be **above** your heart when doing this stance

c) Now, keeping your back straight and firm, hold this position for a while

ATTENTION!

This stance must **not** be done by people with low blood pressure

DID YOU KNOW...

in qi gong, the position of your hands affects your qi? By keeping your hands above your heart, your blood pressure will actually come down. This stance also rids you of those nasty headaches which are a byproduct of high blood pressure

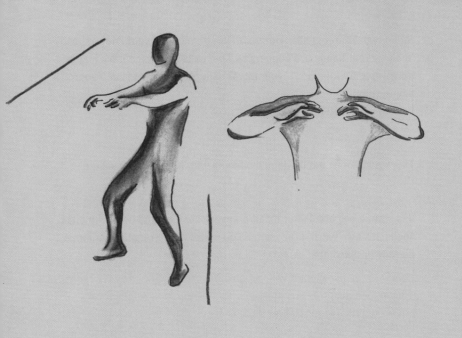

a) Stand with your feet shoulder width apart and bend your knees slightly

b) Imagine your hands are cupping two big balls and place them just in front – but not touching – your lower belly. Remember to keep your elbows open

c) Hold this position for a while

ATTENTION!

This stance must **not** be done by people with high blood pressure

DID YOU KNOW...

this stance will bring your blood pressure back up and help with dizzy spells. It's also worth practising if you suffer from irregular menstrual periods or diarrhoea

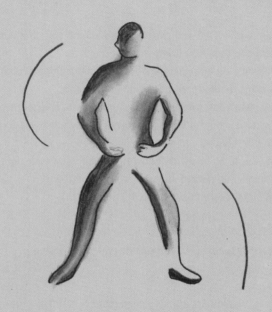

a) Put your left leg forward and your right leg behind you. Keep your weight in the centre and your feet firmly on the ground

b) Position your arms a little distance away from the sides of your body, with your palms facing forward and fingers spread

c) Now gently push your arms forward as though you're scooping water

d) At the same time, your body weight moves with you as you go forwards, bending your left leg as you do so

e) Then push your arms back, shifting your weight onto your right leg, bending it as you do so and straightening your left leg

f) Repeat several times and switch to the other leg

WHAT IT DOES

This stance massages all your muscles and peps you up

DID YOU KNOW...

this stance so resembles the fluid movement of running your hands through water that it is called "Scooping Water" in Chinese?

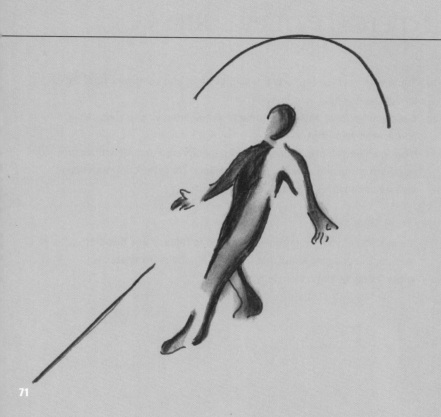

TO FIGHT DEPRESSION

a) Stand with your left leg forward, slightly bent, and keep your right leg straight and behind your body

b) Bend your elbows, raise your arms to shoulder level, cup your palms, and spread your fingers

c) Now imagine you are pushing at an imaginary wall and remember to refrain from looking at red or yellow objects. Try to look at green things instead because it's a lovely calming colour

DID YOU KNOW...

the position of your fingertips is designed to release and disperse tension. Did you also know that the pushing action dissipates your angry thoughts and melancholy?

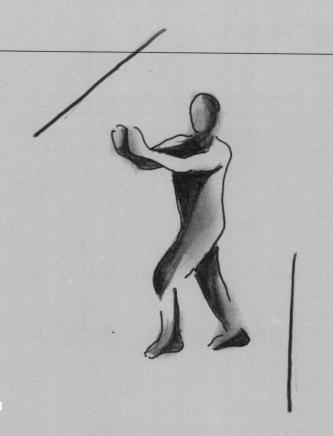

a) Stand with your feet apart, bend your arms – elbows outwards – and raise them to chest level with palms facing the ground and fingers spread
b) Now bend your knees but without moving your arms so that they wind up above your head when you squat. Imagine you're resting them on a high ledge
c) Slowly turn your head to the left, and then to the right, straightening your legs as you do so
d) Return your head to the original position

WHAT IT DOES

This stance stretches and relaxes your muscles especially in the neck

DID YOU KNOW...

the Chinese call this stance Tortoise Coming Out For Air. How apt!

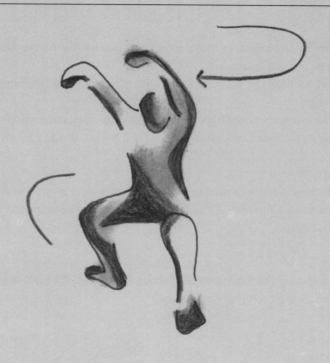

TO ASSUAGE ANGER

a) Assume an imaginary sitting position with your feet apart at shoulder width and your knees bent
b) Put your hands on your hips taking care to ensure your upper body is straight
c) Now rotate your body from the waist in a deep clockwise movement
d) Repeat this exercise 7 times and then do it anti-clockwise 7 times

WHAT IT DOES

Because this stance relaxes your neck and shoulder muscles and aids blood circulation, it's particularly effective for alleviating anxiety and anger

DID YOU KNOW...

you can also do this stance after sitting at your desk for extended periods to loosen your neck muscles

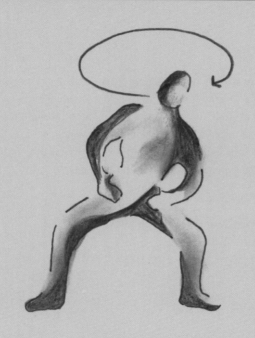

WHEN YOU'RE IN LOVE

A) First Stance

a) Cross your legs and sit in the lotus position
b) Rest the backs of your hands on your thighs, ensuring that your hands look as though they are holding a tennis ball in each palm and your fingers are spread and thumbs facing the sky
c) Remember to keep your elbows out to the side and your eyes open, with your head slightly tilted towards the ground

WHAT IT DOES

Promotes tranquility and calms your beating heart!

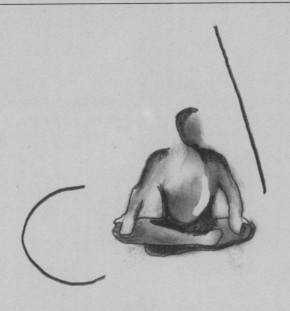

B) Second Stance

a) Cross your legs and sit in the lotus position
b) Rest your hands on your thighs, with the back of one hand resting on the open palm of the other and your thumbs pointing towards the sky
c) Remember to keep your elbows out to the side and your eyes open, with your head slightly tilted to the ground

WHAT IT DOES

Like the first stance, this movement also calms you down when you're all a-flutter

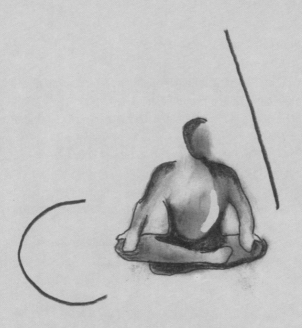

A) First Stance - "The Helicopter"

a) Stand with your feet apart at shoulder width and look straight ahead with your head in the basic qi gong head position
b) Raise your arms above your head and place the backs of your hands on each other
c) Now, keeping your head and legs immobile, turn your body as far as you can to the left and then bring your hands down
e) Return to the original forward position and repeat step (b)
f) Now turn your body the other way, again keeping your head and legs immobile and bring arms down again
h) Repeat from side to side for as long as you like, remembering that the faster you do this stance, the more effective it will be

WHAT IT DOES

This stance is super for toning your waist and arms

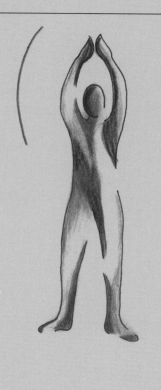

B) Second Stance - "Tiptoes"

a) Stand with your feet apart, on slight tiptoe, keeping your legs straight
b) Lean forward slightly from the hip, with your arms raised above your head at an angle, keeping them straight and fingers spread
c) Hold this position for as long as you can
d) Have a rest and repeat, again staying in position for as long as possible

DID YOU KNOW...

this stance is great for all-over slimming and it also relieves constipation

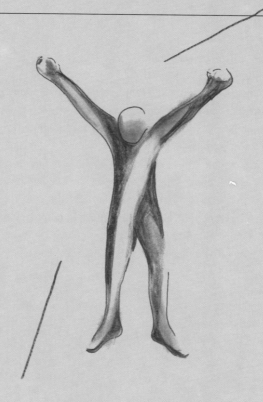

C) Third Stance - "The Woodchopper"

a) Stand with your legs straight and feet apart at shoulder width
b) Take a deep breath and raise your arms high above your head.
   Clasp your hands with your index finger pointing, as though you're
   James Bond aiming a gun
c) Exhale and swing your arms downwards all the way between your
   legs – keeping your hands clasped – so that you wind up bending
   forward from the torso without moving your legs. Imagine you're a
   woodchopper at work and you get the picture, but do remember that
   this stance is more effective when executed quickly
d) Raise your body and arms as in (b), inhaling as you do so, and repeat

DID YOU KNOW...

this exercise is very good for strengthening and toning your tummy

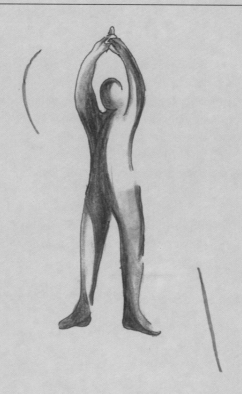

a) Stand on your left leg. Bend your right leg and with your right foot off the ground, make a circular motion with it
b) Ensure that your left leg is slightly bent and your hands are at your sides but away from your body. Your arms should be slightly bent, with palms facing downward, and fingers spread
c) Don't forget - you should use your arms to help you balance
d) Change sides and draw circles with your other leg

WHAT IT DOES

Gets rid of that horrid ironmonger pounding in your head and makes you less of a dullard. No promises if you drink to excess though!

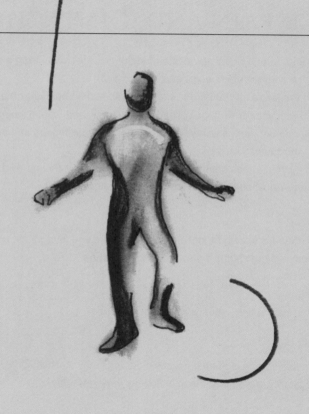

a) With your knees slightly bent, stand about two feet away from a counter or ledge with your legs apart at shoulder width

b) Using the ledge or counter for support (it should be no higher than your chest) rest your arms on it, spread your elbows, and – palms inwards – lightly cup but don't touch your hands. Spread your fingers and make sure your thumbs face the sky

c) Keeping your knees bent, lean forward at a steep angle and hold that position. You should feel the weight in your elbows

WHAT IT DOES

This stance is excellent for relieving backache and joint pains. A handy side benefit is it also cures constipation

ATTENTION!

Do this stance only when a bathroom is nearby!

DID YOU KNOW...

when this stance is done correctly, your legs may start shaking involuntarily, a sign that the qi is flowing very smoothly

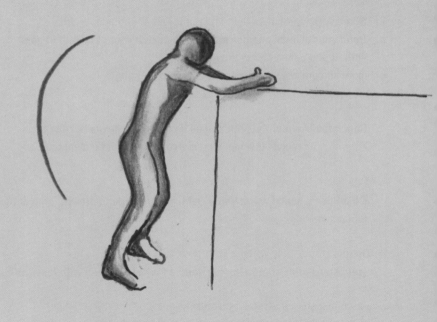

RELIEVING HEADACHES

a) Stand with your knees bent and feet apart at shoulder width
b) Bend your elbows and put your hands next to your ears with fingers spread and palms facing the ground
c) Now tilt your body backwards at a 45-degree angle

WHAT IT DOES

Regulates blood circulation and as as a result relieves headaches. As with stance xvii, this movement also flushes out flu symptoms

HANDY HINT

Do drink a glass of warm water before this stance to prevent dehydration when sweating

DID YOU KNOW...

you can use this stance to cure yourself when you're ill with fever or flu

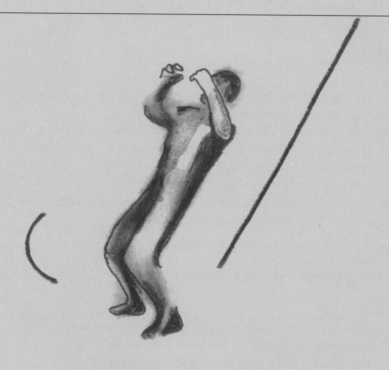

FOR CONSTIPATION

A) First Stance

a) With knees slightly bent, stand about two feet away from a counter or ledge with your legs shoulder width apart

b) Using the ledge or counter for support (it should be no higher than your chest) rest your arms on it, spread your elbows, and – palms inwards – lightly cup but don't touch your hands. Spread your fingers and make sure your thumbs face the sky

c) Keeping your knees bent, lean forward at a steep angle and hold that position. You should feel the weight in your elbows

ATTENTION!

Do this stance only when a bathroom is nearby!

DID YOU KNOW...

when this stance is done correctly, your legs may start shaking involuntarily, a sign that the qi is flowing very smoothly.
This stance is also a great joint and back ache reliever

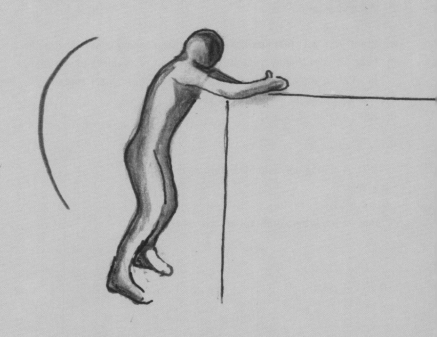

B) Second Stance

a) Stand with your feet apart, on slight tiptoe, keeping your legs straight
b) Lean forward slightly from the hip, with your arms raised above your head at an angle, keeping them straight and your fingers spread
c) Hold this position for as long as you can
d) Have a rest and repeat

ATTENTION!

Do this stance only when a bathroom is nearby!

DID YOU KNOW...

this stance is also great for all-over slimming

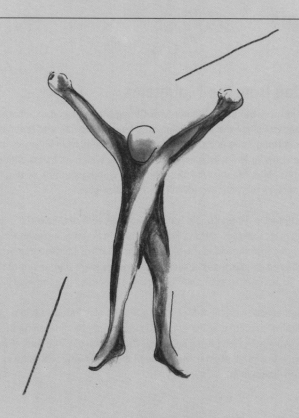

ABOUT MAK CHUNG MAN, QI GONG MASTER

The Man from the Mountains

For the last three decades, Master Mak Chung Man (an avid exponent of qi gong and martial arts since the age of nine) has been practising and teaching qi gong. His clinic in Hong Kong is crowded daily with patients from all walks of life who have come to him with a myriad of ailments which he treats with qi gong massage. At night, Master Mak teaches them qi gong stances so that they can heal themselves with this wonderful spiritual discipline.

Mak Chung Man – Hong Kong's "qi gong ambassador to the world" – was one of the first qi gong masters in Hong Kong to provide qi gong massage. In ancient times, qi gong massage was the exclusive privilege of Chinese emperors because a strong body and enormous reservoirs of energy were demanded of the masseur. To sustain his stamina, Master Mak practises qi gong every day.

A keen and erudite herbalist, Mak Chung Man is also known as "the man from the mountains" because of the time he spends early each morning up in the hills of his village in Hong Kong's Cheung Chau island. With a basket on his back and a hoe in his hand, Master Mak selects the herbs with which he will later concoct his Chinese medicinal potions.

Mak Chung Man's fame as a healer has travelled far and wide and people come to him from all over the world to be treated. In spite of his busy practice, Master Mak still finds time to teach qi gong at the local university because, never possessive of his vast knowledge, Master Mak has always believed that qi gong is not a secret art and therefore should not be shrouded in mystery. Anyone who is interested in qi gong should not be dependent upon a master to do these very simple life-affirming stances. And that, ultimately, is the most eloquent testament to Mak Chung Man, the statuesque healer from the mountains with the bright piercing eyes and kind face who, thanks to his generosity and enthusiasm, has ensured that the ancient art of qi gong will continue to move with the times.